Probiotics: A Step-By-Step Guide To Making Your Own Probiotics For A Healthier Life

Table of Contents

Our gut houses billions of good bacteria that help to regulate the immune system of the body. When these bacteria are altered or destroyed by the use of drugs, antibiotics or by poor lifestyle, they cause diseases and ill health. Probiotics help to repopulate the healthy bacteria present in our gastrointestinal system by adding different strains of flora. This will improve vitality and help to fight off chronic diseases.

What Are Probiotics?

Probiotics are the beneficial bacteria present in the gut, which can promote the production of digestive juices. This will help in the proper functioning of the digestive system. Probiotics are live microorganisms which provide health benefits when administered in the right amounts. There are more than 400 different varieties of bacteria living in the gastrointestinal tract of the humans. These bacteria keep the intestine healthy and aids in proper digestion and absorption of food. They also improve the immunity of the body against various diseases. The most common types of probiotics found in our intestine are L. acidophilus and Bifidobacteria bifidum. These bacteria fight against pathogenic and non- body friendly bacteria like Candida or E-coli. When the probiotics are not present in our gut, there are chances of digestive problems, irritability of the stomach, candidiasis, headaches etc. Lactobacillus acidophilus is one of the strongest probiotic. You can increase the probiotics in your gut by including probiotic foods in your diet and can get the health benefits.

Who All Should Consume Probiotics?

There is no restriction for using the probiotics. They are very effective for people suffering from diarrhea, candidiasis, people who are exposed to toxins in the food, people having a stressful lifestyle and people who have been on antibiotics. Probiotics are highly useful for people in old age to prevent constipation. Probiotics supplement the gastrointestinal bacteria and helps to rebuild the immune system in humans. When you are on antibiotics the good bacteria in your get destroyed along with the pathogenic bad bacteria. So, in order to re-build the colony of the gut bacteria, it is necessary to take probiotics.

Important Probiotic Foods

One of the best known probiotic foods is yogurt. Handmade yoghurts have live cultured bacteria which help in digestion. One of the traditional Japanese probiotic foods is the Miso soup. This made using fermented rye, rice, barley or beans. Sauerkraut is a food made using fermented cabbage. This food helps to reduce allergies they are also rich in Vitamins A, B, C and E. Kefir is another fermented dairy product which is similar to yoghurt. This food is high in probiotic bacteria, such as lactobacilli and bifidus. Kefir is rich in antioxidants and helps to prevent cancer. Kombucha is a fermented tea that contains healthy gut bacteria. Homemade green pickles are an excellent source of probiotic bacteria. Tempeh is probiotic rich soy based grain, which is also a good source of vitamin B12.

The Health Benefits Of Probiotics

Daily intake of probiotics in your diet can fetch you many health benefits. The health benefits of probiotics include

- Enhanced power of immunity- Studies have shown that probiotics regulates the lymphocytes and antibodies responsible for the body immunity and enhances the power to fight diseases.

- Alleviating the negative effect of antibiotics- The probiotics favor the growth of healthy bacteria in the gut, which gets destroyed by the use antibiotics.

- Reduces colon irritation- When colon irritation is caused by the use of certain medicines or after the surgery, the probiotics are extremely helpful in reducing the irritation.

- Better digestion of food- The probiotics stimulate the production of various digestive enzymes helping in better digestion of the food.

- Reduces infections like vaginitis and candidiasis and the occurrence of yeast infections- The probiotic bacteria fights and neutralizes the effect of these bacteria and yeast which causes these infections.

- Reduces the chances of digestive disorders like irritable bowel syndrome, constipation and diarrhea- The probiotics help in the easy transmission of fecal matter through the intestine and prevents constipation. These bacteria also protect the lining of the intestine and prevent IBS.

- Reducing bad breath or Halitosis- Improper digestion or acidity is one of the reasons for bad breath. By providing proper digestion and neutralizing the acidic gastrointestinal juice probiotics prevents bad breath.

- Improved absorption of calcium- The good bacteria in probiotic food help to absorb calcium in a better way

- Reduces intolerance to lactose- Acidophilus bacteria helps to reduce intolerance to lactose present in dairy foods.

- Reducing diarrhea- infant probiotics significantly reduces the rate of diarrhea and diaper rash in babies

- Increasing the ability to synthesize vitamin B

- Reducing the formation of carcinogens- Some forms of probiotics reduces the conversion of bile into carcinogens by increasing the strength of good bacteria in the gut.

Selecting The Probiotics

The markets are flooded with different options of probiotic foods. There are naturally occurring probiotics present in fermented foods, there are regular foods that are enriched with bacterial cultures, probiotics in the indifferent supplement forms such as powders, pills, tablets and capsules, etc. The consumers can easily get confused by these options and they make bad choices while selecting the probiotic. Here are the tips to select probiotic foods

Select Fermented Foods That Contain Probiotics

Fermentation increases the nutritional value of the food and provides your intestine with a host of good bacteria. The list of fermented foods includes yoghurt, tamari, miso, sourdough bread, kefir, sauerkraut and Kombucha.

Do Not Get The Probiotic Enriched Food

The so called probiotic enriched foods are not effective in giving the health benefits of the naturally fermented foods. When the useful bacteria is separated from its natural cultures and are added to processed foods the benefits are very less. Moreover the baking and chilling can destroy most of these good bacteria.

Do Not Opt For Supplements

If you are opting for probiotics to improve your general health it is better to buy- high quality probiotic rich food. If you are aiming to get special health benefits such as treating IBS you need the particular strain of bacteria available in the form of supplements. For this consult a doctor before getting the supplement.

How To Make Probiotics More Effective?

To get the best health benefits from probiotic foods you need to consider certain things about your diet and lifestyle. The probiotics entering the gut need favorable conditions to grow and multiply. The soluble fibers present in our food called pre-biotics are necessary to maintain the probiotics in the gut. This means you will have to increase your fiber food intake to make the probiotics work optimally.

Minimize Exposure To Medications, Alcohol And Other Toxins

Some of the drugs, alcohol and environmental toxins can affect the existence of the good bacteria in the intestine. So reduce the exposure to these damaging items.

Avoid Junk Food

Junk foods and processed food contain certain ingredients which can irritate the gut lining and promotes the growth of bad bacteria in the intestine. These ingredients make it difficult for the good bacteria to thrive in the gut. Replace junk foods with healthy food containing fruits and vegetables and low fat foods.

Probiotics Foods And Drinks

The following is an insight into the different kinds of probiotics foods and drinks that you can easily make in your home to lead a healthier life.

If you are looking to prepare a tasty probiotic beverage, then there is nothing as tasty as home made Kombucha. It is made from tea, sugar and SCOBY (symbiotic culture of bacteria and yeast). Kombucha is a natural beverage that is loaded with probiotics and amino acids. It will help in boosting your immune system and also help in proper functioning of our intestines. It will help in increasing the good bacteria in the gut. If you need to protect and replenish the gut flora, then kombucha beverage is an ideal choice.

Ingredients

- 10 bags of organic green or black tea (green preferred)

- Starter SCOBY and liquid that you can find in the market easily

- A large ceramic or glass container with a wide mouth at the top

- A cooking thermometer

- A light weight cloth napkin or cheesecloth

- Glass storage bottles with tight sealing tops

- Organic sugar, 1 cup for a gallon of water

- A large rubber band

Step By Step Preparing Procedure

1. Add a cup of organic white sugar into the wide mouthed glass container and add tea bags and then fill the container with boiling water. Make sure that you just fill the water halfway of the jar.

2. You should try to use something to suspend the ten green tea bags above the water in the jar.

3. Allow the green tea to brew for about 10 minutes until the color of the water turns into a nice and dark color. Never stir it.

4. Now add cold water to the brewed tea and make sure that you just fill up to 80 percent of the glass jar. You will need some space to add the SCOBY and the starter liquid.

5. Now, you need to cover the wide mouth of the glass jar with the cheesecloth or the think cloth napkin tightly so that it cools down.

6. Once you feel that the tea has cooled down, you need to test the temperature of the tea with a cooking thermometer.

7. As soon as the temperature of tea is below the body temperature of 98.6 degrees, you can add the starter liquid and SCOBY into the jar.

8. It is important for you to make sure that the tea is below body temperature before adding the SCOBY as it is a live bacteria and yeast culture and heat will kill the SCOBY.

9. Now, once again cover the SCOBY added tea with cheesecloth or napkin so that the brew breathes.

10. Store the covered brew in a dark and slightly warm place that is out of reach of small children especially.

11. You can check out the brew after about 12 to 14 days from its preparation date. You can use a syringe to take the brew out of the glass container.

12. You can taste the brew and check if it tastes a bit sweet. If it does not taste a bit sweet, then you need to cover your brew and

leave it alone in the same dark place for a few more days.

13.   A new SCOBY after the fermentation process will be formed on top if the brew and you just need to move the SCOBY to the side to get at the brew.

14.   If you like the taste of the brew, then you can remove the new and the original SCOBY with clean hands.

15.   Now you can put both the SCOBY's in a glass container and cover it. You should never try to put the SCOBY in the fridge.

16.   With the help of a pitcher or a funnel, you can transfer the Kombucha brew into the glass bottles with tight tops.

17.   If you are not going to brew Kombucha again for a month or so, then you can refrigerate your SCOBY.

Lassi is one of the most popular yoghurt based drinks in India. It originated in the state of Punjab and is often considered to be a health drink that helps digestion and also prevents any intestinal problems. Lassi can be prepared with a lot of fruits and vegetables and there is sweet lassi as ell as salt lassi. Most of the people in India prefer sweet lassi and the most popular type of sweet lassi is the sweet mango lassi. It is sure shot favorite of both the young and the old and people who do not like the taste of yoghurt would also love this special mango lassi.

Ingredients (4 Servings)

- 3 cups yoghurt
- 1 cup ripe and fresh mangoes (Alphonso mangoes if possible)
- ½ cup of sugar
- 2 green cardamoms
- Ice cubes

Step By Step Preparation

1. Take 1 cup of cut and ripe mangoes and beat it in a blender to make a good smooth mango puree.

2. Add the yoghurt, sugar and ice cubes along with green cardamoms in the blender with the mango puree and beat on high for two to three minutes.

3. The ice has to be crushed completely and the lassi inside has to be frothy.

4. Now pour the contents from the blender into tall glasses.

5. You can also keep this lassi stored in your refrigerator for up to three days. Make sure that you cover the drink before placing it in the refrigerator.

6. You need to whip it once again in a blender before serving.

Natto is a very popular Japanese probiotic food that is made from fermented soybeans. It is often served with rice. There has to be great care taken when preparing this dish. It is loaded with Vitamin K and is also rich in nattokinase which will help in preventing blood clots as it is a natural blood thinner. Natto can be bought in all popular Asian stores and markets. It is important that you use sterile utensils, cheesecloth, pots and so on when preparing Natto dish.

Ingredients And Things Needed

- 4 cups of soybeans

- One spoonful of Nattomoto powder (sue the same measuring spoon provide in the Natto pack)

- Ceramic or stainless steel pot

- Cheesecloth

- 4 oven proof glass containers that have lids

- A large stainless spoon

Step By Step Preparation

1. Soak the soybeans in water for about 10 to 12 hours. Make sure that you wash the soybeans before soaking. You need to add three parts of water for one part of soybeans.

2. Now drain the soaked water off and now put these beans in a large pot. You need to fill the pot with water and let the soybeans boil in the water for another 9 hours.

3. After boiling you need to drain off the water and put the boiled soybeans in a sterilized pot.

4. Now dissolve one spoon of natto spores from the special spoon into 2 teaspoons of sterilized water.

5. You need to pour the natto spores solution over the beans when the beans are still warm. Now, mix the beans and the natto solution carefully so that they mix well.

6. Now place thin layers of this soaked and natto coated beans in the 4 containers.

7. Cover each of these containers with sterilized cheesecloth and then place the lids of these containers so that the lids sit tightly on top of the containers.

8. Preheat the oven to about 100 degrees and place these covered containers in the oven and allow them to ferment in the oven at 100 degrees for 22 to 24 hours.

9. After the fermentation process for a day, now allow the Natto to cool down for about 2 to 3 hours. Now, you can remove the lid and the cheesecloth and then replace the lid and store the prepared natto in refrigerator for a full day or at least the entire night.

10.   Natto can be served as a breakfast dish in the morning and the remaining Natto will stay fresh and consumable in refrigerator for about 3 to 4 days.

Kefir is another popular probiotic drink that is generally thicker than that of milk. It is made by mixing kefir grains with cow's or goat's milk and then allowing this mixture to ferment for a day. Kefir can be made with milk or with water as well. Milk kefir is a beverage that is made using live bacteria and yeast and can be sued to flavor smoothies, salads and so on. Water kefir is a dairy devoid kefir that is made using sugar and water, juice or even coconut water.

Ingredients For Milk Kefir

- Organic kefir grains

- A glass jar of whole milk

Step By Step Procedure

1. You need to get organic and pure kefir grains to prepare milk kefir. Just place the kefir grains that contain yeast, proteins and bacteria into the glass jar that contains whole milk.

2. Cover the jar with a clean cloth or napkin or cheese cloth and allow the milk to ferment for about a day or two.

3. You need to add approximately a teaspoon full of Kefir grains for 250 ml of milk to prepare the best milk kefir.

4. You will know that the kefir is ready when the milk has turned thicker like yoghurt. You can drink the kefir right way or use it is as a taste enhancing agent. You can store the milk kefir in the fridge for a few days.

Ingredients For Water Kefir Lemonade

- 1 teaspoon of water kefir

- 1/3 or ¼ cup of lemon juice

Step By Step Procedure

1. You need to first prepare a thick lemon juice with water and squeezing out one or two fresh pieces of lemon in the water. Add sugar to taste.

2. Now add the organic water kefir in the lemon juice and stir well so that the kefir and lemon juice combines.

3. You can consume this juice immediately or after refrigeration.

4. If you would like to prepare a carbonated probiotic beverage, then you need to pour the lemonade kefir mixture into airtight bottles.

5. Leave the juice bottles at room temperature for three to four days and then refrigerate it. You can drink the juice once it is chilled.

Sauerruben is nothing but something similar to fermented cabbage and it is usually made with grated turnips. It is not an easily available dish that you can find in the stores. But, sauerruben can be easily made in your home. It is also made with rutabagas and actually the combination of both turnips and rutabagas tastes really good and is the perfect probiotics food that will help in boosting your immunity and metabolism. It is nothing but preparing fermented turnips and fermented rutabagas.

Ingredients

- 5 to 6 large turnips
- 3 to 4 rutabagas
- Sea salt to taste
- Tea towel

Step By Step Preparation

1. Peel and grate the turnips and the rutabagas. You can prepare separate fermented turnips and fermented rutabagas or even mix both of them to prepare a special probiotic food.

2. Now add three tablespoons of sea salt to the grated turnips and rutabagas and mix it well so that the salt evenly spreads and covers the entire grated veggies.

3. The season turnips and rutabaga mixture now should be packed tightly into a heavy duty plastic bucket.

4. Cover the open end of the plastic bucket with a ceramic plate and you need to keep the inside of the bucket airtight. This can be done by placing a heavy glass jar filled with water on top of the ceramic plate.

5. Use a tea towel to cover the entire thing. Place the bucket in a cool land a dark place.

6. The bacteria will be ready to perform the fermentation task when the temperature is about 68 degrees. The higher the temperature the faster will be the work done by the bacteria.

7. Once the turnips ferment after about 4 to 5 days, you can taste the sauerruben everyday. Once you find the fermented turnips to taste really great, you can shift them to a refrigerator to enjoy the same flavor till the last.

a) Fermented Pickles

You do not need to use the artificial vinegar to pickle vegetables. You can easily do this the probiotics way by mixing vegetables like cucumber in a brine of salt and water. This is a natural way of fermenting vegetables and even though you can find these brine pickles to be sold in stores, they are very expensive and hence you can make them very easily in your homes at half the cost.

Ingredients

- 6 to 8 middle finger sized un-waxed cucumbers with the skin

- 2 tablespoons sea salt

- 1 ½ cups of pure water

- 2 garlic cloves, peeled and smashed

- 1 teaspoon of peppercorns

- 6 to 8 fresh dill sprigs

- A wide mouthed glass jar

Step By Step Procedure

1. Wash the cucumbers and cut both the ends of the cucumber tips. You can cut the cucumber into halves or in any shape that you like. It would be tasty if you could cut the cucumbers in pointing finger or middle finger sizes.

2. In a vessel, mix sea salt and the water and allow the salt to completely dissolve in the plain water.

3. Now, in the wide mouthed jar, put 4 sprigs of dill, pepper corns and smashed garlic cloves.

4. Now pack the cucumber in the jar tightly and also add the remaining sprigs of fresh dill.

5. You need to pour the salt mixed water into the jar and make sure that the cucumber is completely submerged with this salt water.

6. Now place the lid on top of the jar and do not seal it completely. Let the jar be placed over the counter top undisturbed at room temperature.

7. You will find after a couple of days that the water has turned cloudy and some air bubbles rise to the top of the water.

8. It will take at least three to ten days for the pickle to be completely done.

9. Start tasting the pickle after the third day and see if it suits your taste and flavor.

10.   Once you find that they are done, you can tighten the lid and store the pickles in the refrigerator. It will stay fresh for about a week.

www.ingramcontent.com/pod-product-compliance
Lightning Source LLC
Chambersburg PA
CBHW071324280526
45788CB00004B/2004